The Body Control Pilates

Pocket Traveller

By Lynne Robinson, Helge Fisher and Paul Massey MCSP

PAN BOOKS

First published 2002 by Pan Books
an imprint of Pan Macmillan Ltd
Pan Macmillan, 20 New Wharf Road,
London N1 9RR
Basingstoke and Oxford
Associated companies throughout
the world
www.panmacmillan.com

ISBN 0 330 49106 7

A CIP catalogue record for this book is
available from the British Library.

Designed and typeset by
Roger Hammond

Printed and bound by Proost, Belgium

9 8 7 6 5 4 3 2 1

Contents

Introduction

TRAVELLING LONG DISTANCE is fast becoming part of modern-day living, for both our business and leisure plans. But any long journey, whether by aeroplane, train, coach or car, upsets our daily rhythms, circulation, digestion and posture. How many times have you arrived home from a two-week holiday feeling you need a two-week holiday? Have you ever turned up for a business meeting abroad knowing full well that you are functioning well below your normal best? And as you climb out of your car after several hours driving, do your neck and shoulders ache, your legs feel stiff and your back feel tight? Whether you are a businessman on a long-haul flight, a taxi driver in a cab or a commuter on the 8.15 to Paddington, the fact is that getting to your destination involves sitting immobile for long periods of time, and can leave you feeling uncomfortable.

The aim of this book is to give you practical advice to ensure that you enjoy your journey and arrive at your destination in peak condition – rested and refreshed. We will be making simple recommendations that anyone can follow, which will help to make the whole travelling experience safer and more comfortable and help you cope more easily in your new environment when you finally arrive.

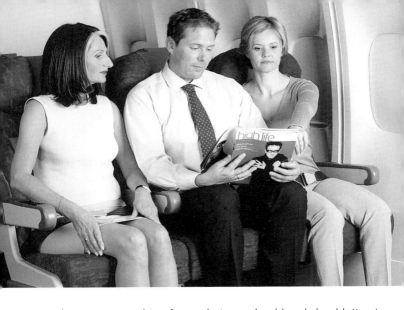

With tips on everything from what you should and shouldn't eat and drink to how to counter jet lag, this pocket book will become as invaluable as your travel guide.

Our main focus, however, is to offer you exercises to do before, during and after your journey. Exercise is a vital part of travel well-being. Our exercises are based on the Body Control Pilates Method, which has a proven track record in many areas of sport, health and fitness. Unique in its approach to body awareness, good movement, postural alignment and core stability, Pilates has helped top athletes, such as those in the England cricket team, to enhance their performance and prevent injuries. We also work in a rehabilitation role with people suffering from back, shoulder, neck and knee problems. This doesn't mean, however, that you need to be injured to do Pilates; many of our clients come to us simply because they want to look and feel great – there is no more effective method of reshaping the body.

We really can, therefore, get you there in better shape!

The short workouts included in this book are designed to:
> **stretch out tight muscles**
> **mobilize joints to keep them flexible**
> **relax parts of the body prone to tension**
> **improve circulation**
> **keep the back supple and strong**

So, whether travelling for business or pleasure, whether you travel just once a year or your job involves travelling frequently, follow the advice below and you should arrive feeling relaxed and ready to enjoy your stay.

Are you fit to travel?

PROBABLY THE FIRST question to ask yourself when thinking about booking a trip is the simplest: 'Am I fit to travel?'

Modern technology has ensured that travel has never been safer or more comfortable. We are getting to our destinations more quickly and, compared with the travelling conditions our ancestors endured, in relative luxury! Nevertheless, the fact remains that travel upsets our normal body patterns and systems so we need a certain level of fitness and good health before we embark on a journey.

If you are at all worried about your fitness to travel then check with your doctor. You should definitely discuss your travel plans with your doctor if you suffer from any medical conditions, or are on long-term medication. Check if you need to take any special precautions.

Deep venous thrombosis (DVT)
Although recently DVT has been much discussed in the media, its dangers are not new. Inappropriately labelled 'economy-class syndrome', DVT is by no means restricted to either economy class or air travel. Sitting for long periods anywhere can increase the risk – you may sit for hours at the theatre or cinema, as well as in a car, on a bus or on a train. Newspapers may blame the amount of space available

in cheaper economy seats as one of the major causes of DVT, but this is misleading – indeed, if susceptible, you may also develop DVT even if you are in business or first class. Much research is being done at present into DVT and, at the same time, there are many conflicting and confusing reports and advice on how to avoid it – ranging from eating chocolate to taking pine-bark supplements.

Let's look first at what DVT is. It occurs when people develop blood clots usually in the deep veins of their legs. Clots may sometimes, although rarely, break away from their original location and travel through the heart to the lungs, blocking vital blood vessels and causing what is known as a pulmonary embolism. This may have serious consequences such as chest pain, shortness of breath and even sudden death.

If you can recognize the symptoms, then DVT can be easily treated. However, it is often difficult to diagnose, so are there symptoms you should look for?

> pain or tenderness in one leg, but not the other
> swelling in one leg
> changes in colour, one leg becoming reddish blue, for example
> increased warmth in one leg
> joint pain

If you have any of these, you should see a doctor immediately. However, you should bear in mind that these symptoms are rarely obvious at the time of prolonged sitting and that it can take days or even weeks before the clot becomes apparent or dangerous. Treatment is aimed at preventing the clot from breaking off and travelling to the lungs, heart or brain. So if you are diagnosed with a DVT you may be admitted to hospital for a few days and receive blood-thinning drugs.

It seems that some of us are more prone to developing DVT than others. According to Dr Patrick Kesteven, consultant haematologist at Newcastle's Freeman Hospital, 10 per cent of the population may have a blood abnormality which acts as a predisposing factor to developing blood clots.

So how do you know if you are at risk?

There are a number of well-known risk factors that may mean you are more susceptible to DVT:

> **You have a previous history of DVT or pulmonary embolism.**
> **You are taking hormone treatment – oral contraceptives or hormone replacement therapies (HRT) containing oestrogen.**
> **A family history of DVT or thrombosis (this includes strokes).**
> **You have had recent surgery.**
> **You are pregnant.**

> You have or have had a malignancy (that is, some cancers).
> You have a genetic blood-clotting abnormality.
> You have had a recent lower-limb injury.
> Some research suggests that there is an added risk if you smoke, are
  obese or have varicose veins.

However, all doctors agree that immobility is a key factor and, therefore, that moving around or exercising is a sensible preventative measure. But how can you safely do this when, if you are travelling by air, the seatbelt sign is on, or, if you are driving, you are stuck in a motorway traffic jam? Don't worry, there are lots of things you can do.

During a flight (or travelling by train or coach)

Follow our advice on pages 54-80, but, in particular:
> Keep moving in your seat as much as possible. Stand up and walk, if
  practical, every couple of hours.
> Do the exercises on pages 56-59. These are designed to make the
  muscles in the legs contract and pump blood back to the heart.
> Avoid alcohol, as it may cause dehydration.
> Drink water for comfort – ideally, take a bottle along with you.
> Wear loose clothing.
> Do not cross your legs.

Some doctors recommend small doses of aspirin, to be taken twenty-four hours before the flight, because aspirin helps to reduce clotting in the blood. However, aspirin has not been shown to reduce travel-related DVT and there are potential problems with taking aspirin, as it is contraindicated in certain medical conditions; if you have stomach ulcers for example. You could check with your doctor before taking aspirin. An alternative is to take pine-bark supplement (pycnogenol).

There is some medical research to support the taking of cod liver oil, which in the long term is claimed to have a similar effect to aspirin in thinning the blood.

There has also been some recent research to suggest that wearing graduated compression stockings will help reduce the formation of travel-related blood clots. If you are concerned, or if you are in the high-risk groups, then ask your doctor's advice on wearing compression hosiery. They should be properly fitted.

Driving
Stop and walk around at least every two hours. Not only will this get your circulation going but it will also help to keep you alert.

If you are stuck in a traffic jam, try the seated exercises on pages 54-63.

When you're on a plane you can happily doze off, but in a car you obviously need to stay awake at the wheel! So, if you feel sleepy, stop driving, drink a caffeinated drink such as coffee or cola, and take a short nap before driving on. If you do this try to drink plenty of water as well. In any case, drinking plenty of water is a good idea.

You should wear loose clothing on the journey and consider other measures (see above).

Pre-trip advice

Whether on a long or short trip, there are a few simple things that you can do before you travel to ensure that your journey is stress-free and to help you arrive feeling fantastic.

If you are flying and anxious to avoid jet lag – and you have the freedom to choose which direction you fly in – you should bear in mind that flying westwards is less likely to upset your body clock. Why? Even though our day is twenty-four hours long, our internal body clock prefers a day to be a little longer. Flying westward extends your day whereas flying eastward shrinks it. See pages 82-84 for other tips on combating jet lag.

Leave plenty of time to get to the airport, rail or coach station. Nothing is guaranteed to stress you as much as being late for check-in!

Getting medical advice

It makes good sense to discuss your travel plans with your GP or hospital specialist, especially if you suffer from a medical condition or are taking long-term medication. You can also get a lot of information from the internet but it is no substitute for a consultation with your travel medicine adviser. Do bear in mind that if vaccinations are required, some courses of injections take several weeks to complete, so do not leave it to the last minute!

If you do need to take medication with you, remember to pack it in your hand luggage. Make sure you have enough for the whole trip, plus extra, in case of delays.

Packing

Pack light. Remember that you will have to lift your suitcases at some point in your journey, in and out of a taxi for example or on and off the baggage carousel.

You will also have to lift your hand luggage into the overhead lockers or train or coach racks, so ensure that your hand baggage is as light as possible. The aircrew-type cases with wheels attached are ideal, but be aware that with this type of luggage you are twisting and pulling at the same time and this places considerable strain on the spine. When wheeling these cases, you should alternate the side from which you pull the case, or, better still, if possible push it. If you are driving and have to lift your suitcases onto a roof rack then follow the advice given below on lifting safely.

Size restrictions apply on all airlines and for some coach operators. The International Air Transport Association's (IATA) recommendation is that cabin luggage should not exceed 115 centimetres in dimension, calculated by adding the length, height and depth measurements of the bag. Charter airlines may only accept a lower maximum size, so always check your carrier's regulations before you fly. Please note that many airlines have changed their regulations since the events of September 11th, 2001 – this includes passengers not being allowed to pack any sharp objects in hand baggage.

If you need a lumbar roll or an inflatable neck support, or if you like to use ear plugs and/or eyeshades, put them somewhere easily accessible.

You may want to take some toiletries to freshen up before you depart and also a change of underwear – have them somewhere to hand.

If you are flying, take a moisturizer with you, as your skin will feel dry on board. When you pack your on-board bathroom bag, think about your time of arrival. If you are travelling to a hot climate and are arriving at midday, you may need a sunscreen handy. If you arrive at night, mosquito repellent may be needed.

Pack some entertainment – lightweight games, paperback books, music etc.

When you buy luggage, choose a suitcase that is not too heavy before it is filled. The normal airline limit for a packed suitcase is in the region of 20 kilograms, but try to stay below this. Hard-shell suitcases will protect your belongings better than those with soft casings.

If you have back problems, spread your packing over several days and place your suitcase on a surface at a height that means you avoid bending forward repeatedly.

Meals

Keep your pre-journey meals light. It is also wise to avoid heavily spiced food. If flying, avoid carbonated drinks and restrict your intake of caffeine via tea, coffee and sodas.

Clothing

Try to wear layers of clothes to allow for changes of temperature. Clothes should be loose fitting and have an elasticated waist for comfort as your abdomen may swell during a flight. If you want to arrive looking smart, if possible choose fabrics that are non-crease. Your feet may also swell during a flight, so choose shoes that slip on and off easily and are not too tight – you want to be able to get them on again at the other end! Take an extra pair of socks in case your feet get cold and don't forget your support socks or stockings if you choose to use them – see page 11.

Lifting and carrying

Lifting is potentially the most dangerous action for back-pain sufferers, especially if you combine it with twisting and bending. Good technique is very important to prevent back problems, but you must also allow your back to heal if it is strained or damaged already.

In an ideal world, you should avoid lifting heavy loads completely if your back is fragile. If you cannot avoid doing so, at least take note of the following advice:

> Where possible, take the time to divide the load. It may take a little longer to complete the task, but it is better than harming your back.
> Do not be afraid to ask someone to help you – an extra pair of hands will lighten the load.
> Stop before you lift and note how heavy the load really is. You need to be aware of the weight of the object that you are about to lift so that your body is prepared.
> Stand as close as possible to the load, and have your feet on either side of it with one foot slightly in front of the other (as if you were taking a step).
> Bend at the knee and hip so that you squat down.
> Keep your back long and strongly supported by zipping up and hollowing – see page 24.
> Keep your body close to the load, using the handles or placing one hand under the object with the other on top.

> As you lift, make sure you keep the
  load close to your body. The further
  away you hold the load, the more you
  are straining your back!

> Lean forward and, while maintaining a
  long back, straighten your knees and
  hips.
> When lowering the load, reverse the above advice.
> Avoid lifting and twisting at the same time. Lift first and then rotate the
  whole of your trunk round to where you want to go.
> Avoid carrying a heavy load on one side of your body, try to divide it into
  equal weights.

The eight principles of the

Body Control Pilates Method

THE EXERCISES IN this book have their origins in the work of Joseph
Pilates (1880–1967). Well-proven for over eighty years, they also
incorporate the latest techniques in both mental and physical training
and offer complete body conditioning.

The programme targets the key postural muscles, building
strength from within, by stabilizing the torso. The body is gently

realigned and reshaped, the muscles balanced, so that the whole body moves efficiently. By bringing together body and mind and heightening body awareness, Pilates literally teaches you to be in control of your body, allowing you to handle stress more effectively and to achieve relaxation more easily.

All the exercises in this book are built around the following eight principles.

> Relaxation
> Concentration
> Alignment

> Breathing
> Centring
> Co-ordination

> Flowing movements
> Stamina

Prolonged, seated immobility may put you at risk from developing DVT and can exacerbate exisiting injuries, especially back, neck and knee problems.

Body Control Pilates with its emphasis on good postural alignment, strengthening the deep abdominals and the back muscles, and promoting normal movement patterns is the ideal exercise programme to look after your health in transit. However, there are certain skills which you need to master before you try the main programmes. Ensure that you study and practice the exercises on pages 20-29 before attempting those in the rest of the book.

Body Control Pilates

The basic exercises

Before you start
> The exercises should ideally be done on a padded mat.
> Wear something warm and comfortable which allows free movement.
> Barefoot is best, socks otherwise.
> For some of the exercises you may need a firm flat pillow or a folded
  towel, a larger plump pillow, a long scarf and a tennis ball.

Please do not exercise if
> You are feeling unwell.
> You have just eaten a meal.
> You have a bad hangover.
> You have taken painkillers, as they will mask any warning pains.

If you are undergoing medical treatment, are pregnant or injured,
please consult your medical practitioner before exercising. It is always
advisable, in any case, to consult your doctor before taking up a new
exercise regime.

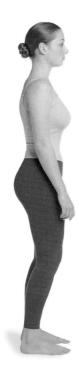

Checking your Alignment

Always take a moment to check that your body is correctly aligned before you start an exercise. Here is a checklist to help:

> Think of the top of the head lengthening away from the tailbone.
> Is my neck tense? Keep your neck released and soft. The back of the neck stays long. When lying down, you may prefer to place a firm flat pillow under your head so that your chin is parallel to the floor.
> Where are my shoulders? Hopefully not up round your ears! Keep the shoulder blades down into your back, with a nice big gap between your ears and the shoulders.
> Is my spine lengthened, but still with its natural curves?
> Is my pelvis in neutral? See page 22.
> Where are my feet? Don't forget them. If they are wrongly placed it will affect your knees, hips and back. Usually, they should be hip-width apart and parallel. Watch that they do not roll in or out!

The Relaxation Position

Lie with your knees bent, your feet in line with your hips, your toes parallel. Your heels are in line with the centre of your buttocks. Your chin should be parallel to the floor so place a firm, flat pillow under your head if necessary. Place your hands on your abdomen to check that your pelvis is in neutral (see below). Allow your whole back to widen and lengthen.

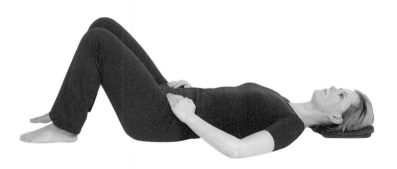

The Position of the Pelvis and Spine

If you exercise with the pelvis and the spine wrongly positioned, you run the risk of creating muscle imbalances and stressing the spine itself. You should aim to have your pelvis and spine in their natural, neutral positions. Imagine a compass has been placed on your pelvis.

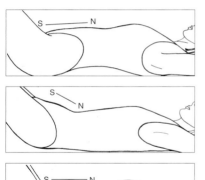

Tilted to south.
The back is overarched.

Tilted to north.
The lumbar curve is lost.

Neutral.
The correct position. The curves of the spine are maintained and the sacrum rests squarely on the mat. The tailbone is down.

Breathing the Pilates Way

In Pilates we use lateral, thoracic breathing for all exercises. This entails breathing into the lower ribcage and back to make maximum use of lung capacity. The increased oxygen intake replenishes the body and the action itself creates greater flexibility in the upper body.

To learn lateral breathing you may sit, stand or kneel with your pelvis in neutral and the spine lengthened.

Equipment
A scarf.

Action
> Wrap a scarf around your lower ribcage, cross the ends over in front of you and pull on them a little to feel where you are working. The idea is to breathe into the scarf, directing the breath into your sides and back, but keeping the shoulders down and relaxed, and the neck calm. The ribs expand as you inhale and close down as you exhale.
> Repeat six times, but do not over-breathe or you may feel dizzy. Breathe softly in a relaxed way.

Creating a Strong Centre

Nearly all Pilates exercises involve engaging the deep postural muscles to protect the spine as you exercise. This is called stabilizing or centring and creates a girdle of strength from which to move.

To find these deep muscles, adopt the Starting Position opposite.

Starting Position
> Come on to all fours, your hands beneath your shoulders, your knees beneath your hips.
> Look straight down at the floor; the back of the neck stays long, the elbows soft, the spine maintaining its natural, neutral curve. Imagine that you have a small puddle of water cradled in the base of your spine.

Action

> Breathe in wide to prepare, and lengthen through the spine.
> Breathe out, engage the muscles of your pelvic floor (as if you are trying not to pass water) and hollow your lower abdominals back to the spine. Do not move the pelvis or spine. Keep the action low and gentle.
> Now breathe normally while keeping the muscles engaged – this takes practice!
> Think of it as an internal zip which begins underneath and zips up and in to hold your lower abdominal contents in place, just like zipping up your trousers – we call this zipping up and hollowing.

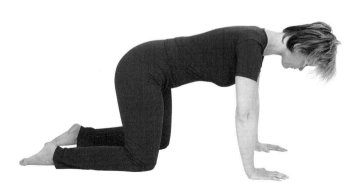

The Upper Body

In Pilates, you must think about the whole body with every exercise, so moving the upper body well is vital. The following exercises help you to locate the muscles that set the shoulder blades down into the back.

The Dart

Equipment
Two small flat pillows (optional).

Starting Position
> Lie on your front – place a flat pillow under your forehead to allow you to breathe more easily if you wish.
> If it's more comfortable, you may place a small pillow underneath your stomach.
> Have your arms down by your sides with your palms facing your body.

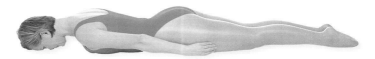

> Your neck is long.
> Your legs are relaxed with the toes touching and the heels apart.

Action
> Breathe in wide and lengthen through the spine. Tuck your chin in gently.
> Breathe out, zip up and hollow, and pull your shoulder blades down into your back, bringing the upper body slightly off the floor. At the same time, squeeze your inner thighs together, and bring your heels together.
> Reach your fingers away from you down towards your feet. The top of your head stays lengthening away from you.
> Keep looking straight down at the floor. Do not tip your head back.
> Breathe in and lengthen from the top of the head to the tailbone.
> Breathe out and release.
> Repeat six times, keeping your feet on the floor.

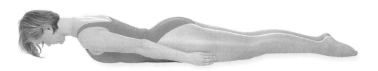

Floating Arms

Starting Position
> Stand correctly – see page 23.
> Place your right hand on top
  of your left shoulder, this is to
  check that the muscle there
  stays relaxed, while the mid-
  back muscles below your
  shoulder blades work to set
  the shoulder blades down
  into your back.

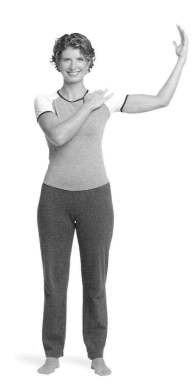

Action
> Breathe in wide, and lengthen up through the spine.
> Breathe out, zip up and hollow, and slowly move the hand and
  arm upwards and sideways, reaching wide out of the shoulder
  blades like a bird's wing. Think of the hand as leading the arm, the
  arm following the hand as it floats upwards.
> Rotate the arm, so that the palm opens to the ceiling as the arm
  reaches shoulder level.
> Try to keep the upper part of the shoulder under your left hand
  still and both shoulder blades dropping down into your back for as
  long as possible.
> Keep your body central.
> Breathe in as you lower the arm to your side.
> Repeat three times with each arm.

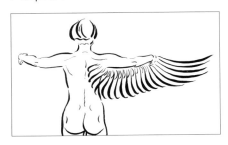

Pre-trip exercises

The following short programme has been specially designed to balance your body in preparation for the journey ahead.

Leg Slides

This exercise teaches you how to keep the pelvis stable while moving the legs.

Starting Position
Lie in the Relaxation
Position.

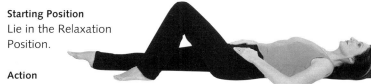

Action
> Breathe in
  wide and full to prepare.
> Breathe out, zip up and hollow, and slide one leg away along the
  floor, keeping the lower abdominals scooped. The pelvis stays still,
  stable and in neutral.
> Breathe in, then out, still zipped as you return the leg to the bent
  position, trying to keep the stomach hollow.
> Repeat five times with each leg.

Floating Arms in Lying

This exercise teaches good upper-body movement. Remember what you learnt in the standing version on page 28.

Starting Position
Lie in the Relaxation
Position.

Action
> Breathe in
  wide into
  your lower ribcage to prepare.
> Breathe out, zip up and hollow, and slowly move one arm back as if to touch the floor – like a backstroke movement. You may not be able to touch the floor comfortably so only move the arm as far as you are happy to do so. Do not force it, keep it soft and open, the elbow bent.
> The shoulder blade stays down into your back. The ribs stay calm and do not flare up. Do not allow the back to arch at all.
> Breathe in as you return the arm to your side.
> Repeat five times with each arm.

31

The Starfish

Starting position
Lie in the Relaxation Position, but with your arms by your side.

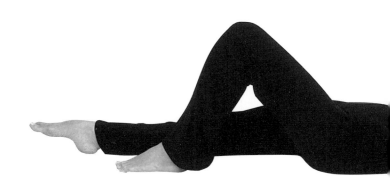

Action

> Breathe in wide and full to prepare.
> Breathe out, zip up and hollow, slide the right leg away along the floor, in line with your hips, and take the left arm above you in a backstroke movement.
> Keep the pelvis completely neutral, stable and still and the stomach muscles engaged.
> Keep a sense of width and openness in the upper body and shoulders, and try to keep the shoulder blades down into your back and the ribs calm.
> Breathe in, still zipped, and return the limbs to the Starting Position.
> Repeat five times, alternating arms and legs.

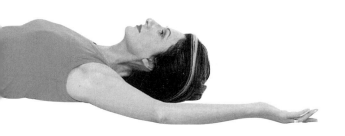

Hip Rolls

This exercise works the waist muscles and keeps the spine flexible.

Warning: please take advice if you have a disc-related injury.

Optional equipment
A tennis ball.

Starting Position
> Lie in the Relaxation Position, but with the feet together. If you
  have a tennis ball, put it between the knees.

> Place your arms out to the sides in a line
  with your shoulders, your palms facing up.

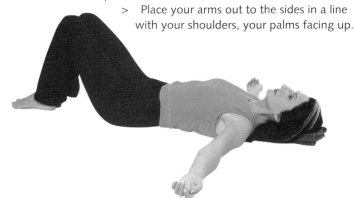

Action

> Breathe in wide and full.
> Breathe out, and zip up and hollow. Staying zipped throughout,
  roll your head in one direction, your knees in the other. Only roll a
  little way to start with – you can go further each time as long as it
  is comfortable. Keep your opposite shoulder down on the floor.
  Try to keep your knees together, the ball still and the legs in line.
> Breathe in wide, then breathe out. Use your strong centre to bring
  the knees and head back to the Starting Position.
> Repeat eight times in each direction.

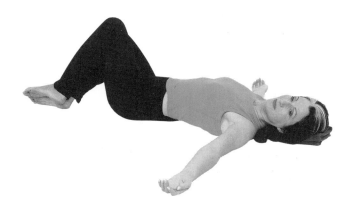

Hamstring Stretch

Warning: if you suffer from sciatica or disc-related problems, please take advice before trying this exercise.

Equipment
A long scarf or a stretch band.

Starting Position
> Lie in the Relaxation Position.
> Put the scarf over your foot, then return to the neutral spine and pelvis position. Hold the scarf from underneath so that your upper body stays open and relaxed.

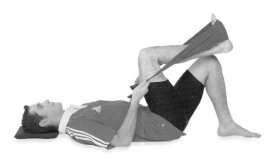

Action

> Breathe in wide and full.
> Breathe out, zip up and hollow and stay zipped throughout.
> Slowly straighten the leg into the air. Keep the foot relaxed – think of lengthening through the heel. Make sure that the leg stays parallel, the kneecap facing you in a line with your hip. Keep your tailbone down on the floor. The pelvis stays neutral.
> Breathing normally, hold the stretch for a count of about 30 seconds or until you feel the muscles at the back of your thigh release. Relax the leg by gently bending it again.
> Repeat three times with each leg, constantly checking that your tailbone stays down and your pelvis stays in neutral.

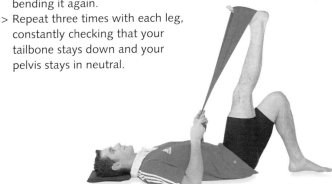

Side-lying Quadriceps Stretch

This will help to stretch out the muscles that run down the front of the thigh. These tend to shorten when you sit for long periods of time.

Warning: please take advice if you have a knee injury.

Optional equipment
A scarf or a stretch band and a pillow.

Starting Position
> Lie on your side with your head resting on your extended arm (you may like to put a flat pillow between your head and your arm to keep your neck in line).
> Curl your knees up at a right angle to your body.
> Your back should be in a 'straight' line, but with its natural curve.
> Stack all your bones up on top of each other – foot over foot, knee over knee, hip over hip and shoulder over shoulder.

Action

> Breathe in wide and full.
> Breathe out, zip up and hollow. Staying zipped throughout the exercise, bend the knee of your upper leg towards your chest, taking hold of the front of the ankle if you can reach it. You may need to use a scarf.
> Breathe in, then out, and slowly take the leg back in a line with your torso to stretch the front of the thigh. Do not arch the back, keep the tailbone and the knee lengthening away from the top of the head.
> Breathe normally as you wait for the muscle to release (about 30 seconds).
> Keep working the waist, which stays slightly lifted from the floor, keeping the length in the trunk.
> Slowly release by bringing the leg back in front of you.
> Repeat three times on each side, keeping the leg at hip height.

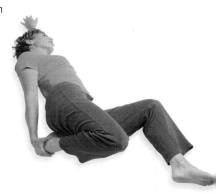

The Corkscrew

Why is it called the corkscrew? Imagine the type of corkscrew where as the arms are brought down the cork pops up – this is like your head coming up as your arms descend.

Starting Position
Stand correctly – see page 20.

Action

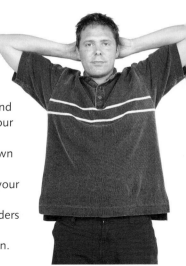

> Breathe in wide, and lengthen up through the spine.
> Breathe out, zip up and hollow and stay zipped throughout. Allow your arms to float upwards. Think of dropping the shoulder blades down into your back as the arms rise.
> Clasp your hands lightly behind your head.
> Breathe in, and shrug your shoulders up to your ears.
> Breathe out, and drop them down.

> Breathe in, and gently bring your elbows back a little – you should still be able to see them. The shoulder blades move together. Do not allow your back to arch.

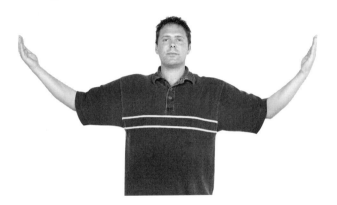

> Breathe out as you release your hands and bring them down by your sides. Open the shoulders wide and engage the muscles beneath your shoulder blades. As you do so think of allowing your head, neck and spine to lengthen up as the arms come down. Think of that corkscrew!
> Repeat five times.

Roll Downs

These will promote flexibility in
your back.

**Warning: please take advice if you have a
back problem.**

Starting Position
> Stand about 45 cm away from a wall,
  facing away from it.
> Lean back into the wall and bend the
  knees (see photo). Your feet should be
  hip-width apart and parallel.
> Your pelvis is in neutral.
> Your head is away from the wall.

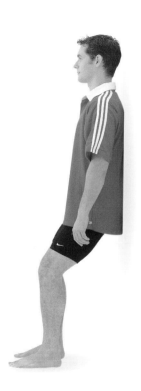

Action

> Breathe in wide and lengthen up through the spine.
> Breathe out, zip up and hollow. Staying zipped throughout, drop your chin on to your chest and start to roll forward, peeling the spine off the wall bone by bone. Release your neck and shoulders. Stay central.
> Breathe in, then out, and drop your tailbone down, rotating your pelvis backwards as you slowly come up the wall, rolling back up through the spine bone by bone, bringing your head up last.
> As you roll back up, think of rebuilding the spinal column, stacking each vertebra on top of the other to lengthen out the spine.
> Repeat six times.

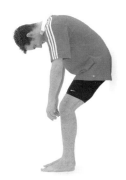

When you have mastered this version, you can try the exercise free-standing. Stand correctly, but leave your knees bent throughout.

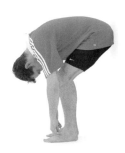

The Diamond Press

As you are going to follow this exercise with the Rest Position, have a plump pillow ready to hand.

Starting Position
> Lie on your front with your feet hip-width apart and parallel.
> Create a diamond shape with your arms by placing your fingertips together just above your forehead. Your elbows are open, your shoulder blades relaxed.

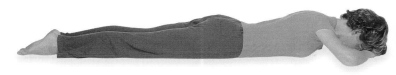

Action

> Breathe in wide and full.
> Breathe out, zip up and hollow and stay zipped throughout. Draw the shoulder blades down towards the small of your back. Gently tuck your chin forward as if holding a ripe peach, and raise your upper body about 4–5 cm off the floor. Stay looking down at the floor, keeping the back of the neck long. Imagine a cord pulling you from the top of your head.
> Breathe in and hold the position. Keep the lower stomach lifted. The ribs stay on the floor.
> Breathe out, and slowly lower back down. Keep lengthening through the spine.
> Repeat six times.

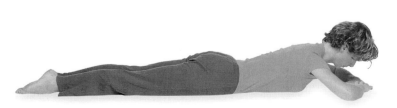

Rest Position

Great for stretching out the lower back.

Warning: please take advice if you have knee problems.

Equipment
A plump pillow.

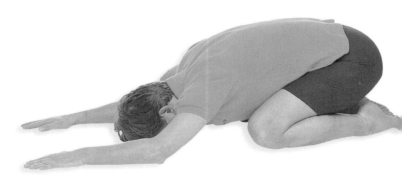

Action

> When you have finished the Diamond Press, come up on to all fours. Bring your feet together, but leave your knees apart.

> Slowly come back to sit on your heels. Place the pillow underneath your knees so as not to compress them.

> Hopefully, you will be able to rest your forehead on the floor, but do not over-reach, stay within your comfort range.

> Relax into this position – focus on breathing into your back.

> Take ten breaths in this position.

To come out of the Rest position

> As you breathe out, zip up and hollow, and slowly unfurl, rebuilding the spine bone by bone, bringing your head up last (as for Roll Downs, page 42).

Well Being

OVER THE YEARS British Airways has accumulated a great deal of knowledge and experience about the effects of air travel on the body. The Well Being programme was first launched in 1993 and offers a range of measures to enhance passenger comfort and awareness. The programme is continuously growing through our work with experts in a range of fields and is designed to enhance your entire journey experience, from before your flight right through to after you arrive.

Pre-flight, passengers receive 'The Healthy Journey', a leaflet with simple advice and suggestions to assist them in their journey which is sent out in every ticket wallet. British Airways also provides a Passenger Medical Clearance Unit, Central London Travel Clinics, as well as a series of health pages on British Airways' website at www.britishairways.com/health.

On board, the programme includes exercises and advice, which have been developed in conjunction with Body Control Pilates. These exclusive exercises were designed specifically for use in the aircraft cabin. They are featured in our in-flight magazine, *High Life*, and as part of the Well Being video. *High Life* also contains monthly articles on topical Well Being issues.

In-flight we also offer a Well Being audio channel, healthy choice menu options, and amenity bags.

For eligible passengers there are departure and arrival lounges, including Molton Brown Travel Spas, available at London Heathrow Airport, which offer a range of complimentary massage treatments and a relaxing environment to revitalize after a long flight.

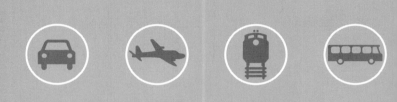

In-flight exercises and advice

THE FOLLOWING ADVICE refers to air travel but much is also relevant to travelling on trains or coaches.

Checking in

> When you arrive at the airport or station, use a trolley to carry your baggage.
> Remember the advice on how to lift your suitcases safely on pages 16-17.
> While you are waiting to depart, try to walk round the departure lounge or platform as much as possible. You'll soon be spending plenty of time sitting. Don't forget to listen for your flight or platform number to be called and keep an eye on the departure board!

On board

> Take care when placing your cabin baggage in the overhead lockers or the overhead racks. Remember your lifting advice.
> Try to keep the area around your feet as free as possible so that you can stretch your legs.
> When flying, don't forget to use your lumbar or neck support if you need it but wait until the aircraft is airborne before inflating your neck support and take care not to over inflate it.
> Use a neck roll when you decide to sleep.
> Use a blanket, as your temperature will drop as you sleep.
> If you have trouble getting to sleep, tune into the on-board 'relaxation' channel, if available, or listen to your own relaxation tape.
> Talk yourself through some simple relaxation techniques.
> Before you sleep, read a book that will relax rather than excite you!
> If you find noise distracting, use ear plugs.
> If you find light distracting, use eyeshades.
> If you wear contact lenses, take them out as soon as you can, as your eyes dry out in the air – and, hopefully, you will be sleeping for some of the journey.
> Eat lightly. A heavy meal may make you feel uncomfortable, so go for the light bite instead.
> Avoid alcohol if you can or, at least, go easy. No more than two glasses of wine.

- > Avoid fizzy drinks (save the champagne for when you arrive!).
- > Drink lots of still, not sparkling, water. Little and often is best.
- > Avoid, or go easy on, the tea, coffee and sodas as the caffeine will keep you awake and may dehydrate you.
- > Plan your journey, so that you can enjoy the meal and the entertainment but also have plenty of time to rest.
- > Sleep as often as you can – even a short nap will help with jet lag.
- > Keep your seat belt fastened whenever you are sitting, but it should not be too tight. Fasten the seat belt over the blanket when you are asleep so that the crew do not have to disturb you.
- > Be a mover – try not to sit still for too long. When convenient, when the aisles are clear and the seat-belt signs are off, stand up and stretch your legs and carry out the following exercises as often as you can, or at least every couple of hours.

In-flight exercise programme

Sit right

As you relax back into your seat, think about how you are sitting.

> Try to keep the natural curves of your spine by placing a small pillow (or a lumbar roll) in the hollow of your lower back.
> Try not to cross your legs. This will help your back and your circulation. If you must cross your legs, alternate them frequently.
> Sit tall. Avoid compressing your spine by sitting with your weight evenly balanced on both buttocks. Lengthen up through the top of your head. Keep your shoulders relaxed and open.
> Locate the deep abdominals that support your spine. Breathe in wide into your sides. As you breathe out, gently zip up the pelvic floor and hollow your lower abdominals back towards your spine. Breathe normally keeping the abdominals 'scooped'.
> Try to stay zipped while you practise the exercises, always remembering to keep breathing!

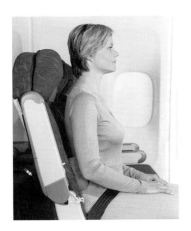

Correct

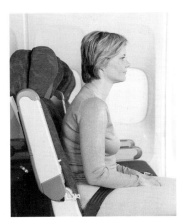

Incorrect

55

Pillow Squeeze in Sitting

Aim
This exercise will work your inner thigh muscles.

Starting Position
> Follow all the directions for sitting well, but this time place the pillow between your knees.
> Have your feet together and parallel.

Action
> Breathe in wide and full, and lengthen up through the spine.
> Breathe out, zip up and hollow, and gently squeeze your pillow between your knees. Keep your feet on the floor and keep the natural curve in your back.
> Breathe normally as you squeeze for a count of ten before releasing.
> Repeat six times.

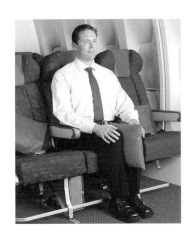

Ankle Circles

Aim
This is a lovely exercise to prevent your ankles from becoming stiff.

Starting position
Sit tall in your seat.

Action
> Place your pillow under your
  right thigh just above the knee,
  keeping your weight even.
> Now circle your right foot
  round, keeping the whole leg
  as still as possible, rotating
  from the ankle joint.
> Make ten circles in each
  direction with each foot.

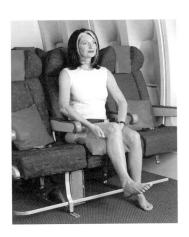

Calf exercise

This exercise is designed to work the deep calf muscles.

Starting Position
> Still sitting tall, take your foot back underneath the seat a little,
>   keeping it in a line with your knee and hip.

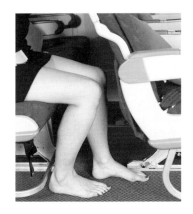

Action

> Keeping the foot flat, push the toes and ball of your foot into the floor, hold for a count of five, then release.
> Now push your heel into the floor for a count of five, release.
> Repeat these two actions with the knee at a right angle and with the leg stretched out a little, again in a line with the knee and hip. You should feel the work deep in your calf.

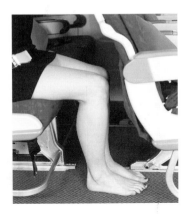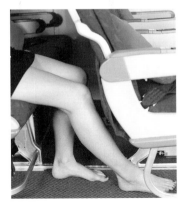

Shoulder Circles

Perfect for releasing tension in the shoulders.

Starting Position
> Sit tall, following all the directions on page 54-5.

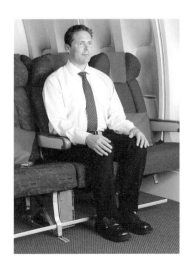

Action

> Move forward a little on your seat.
> Bring your shoulders up towards your ears, then circle them back downwards. Imagine that you have pencils on the tips of your shoulders and that you have to draw big circles.
> Repeat six times, then lift the shoulders towards your ears and drop them back down six times.

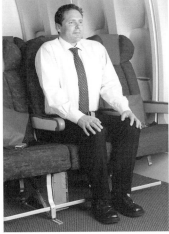

Neck Rolls

For releasing tension in the neck.

Starting Position
> Sit back in your seat.
> If your seat has a headrest, flatten it out.

Action
> Gently and slowly allow your head to roll to one side – do not force it – then roll back through the centre and to the other side.
> Try to keep the back of your neck long and your shoulders relaxed.
> Repeat several times.

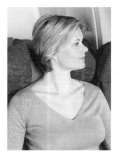 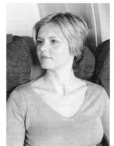

Shoulder Stretch

For stretching out the arms and shoulder area.

Starting Position
> Sit tall in your seat.

Action
> Interlace your fingers.
> Reach your arms above you and stretch away, turning your palms away from you towards the ceiling.
> Do not take your arms behind your head.
> Think of your shoulder blades moving down as you reach up.
> Hold the stretch for three wide breaths.
> Repeat five times.

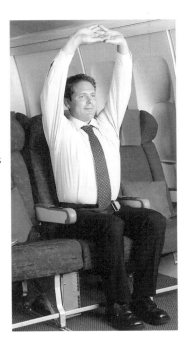

Walking on the Spot

Starting Position
> Hold on to the back of a seat or the cabin wall.
> Stand tall with your feet hip-width apart.

Action
> Start to walk on the spot. Come up on to the balls of both feet, then lower one heel down, staying on the ball of the other foot; that knee bends slightly (check it is bent directly over the centre of your foot).
> Then, change legs, transferring your weight but not wiggling your hips.
> Keep lengthening up, up, up and keep the waist long.
> Continue walking on the spot for a couple of minutes.

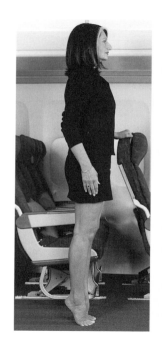

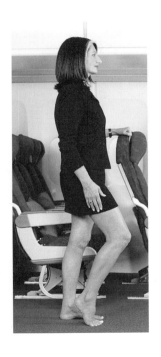 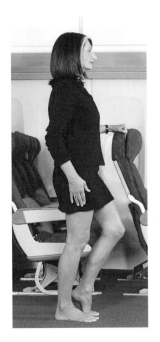

Up and Down

Aim

This exercise works the deep calf muscles.

Starting Position
> Stand tall with your feet parallel, hip-width apart.
> Think about good alignment throughout the body.
> Breathe normally.

Action
> Come up on to your toes, trying not to tip forward. Think of going straight up.
> Continue to think tall as you lower your heels back down. Imagine the top of your head stays up.

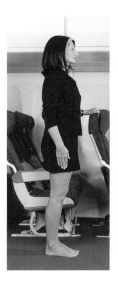

> Bend your knees, so that they come directly over the centre of each foot. Your heels should stay down and your feet should not roll in or out.

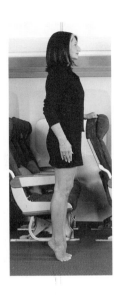 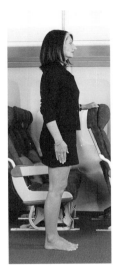 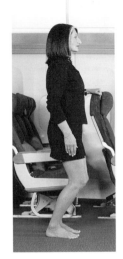

> Try not to stick your bottom out or tuck it under.
> Slowly straighten the leg to return to the Starting Position.
> Repeat ten times.

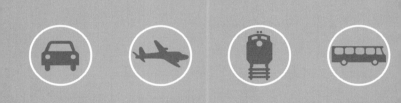

In-transit exercises

IT IS NOT always easy to stand up during a flight, a train or a coach journey (unless you are commuting!), but as soon as you have the opportunity to stretch your legs – if, for example, you are in transit or when you arrive at your destination – do so. Try the following stretches – they will feel blissful after having been sitting for so long. Alternatively, do them as soon as you arrive in your hotel room or get back home.

If you haven't already done Walking on the Spot (page 64) or Up and Down (page 66), then do them first.

Standing Quadriceps Stretch

This is a complementary stretch to the Side-lying Quadriceps Stretch on page 38. As always, alignment is crucial so do not allow the back to arch.

Warning: please take advice if you have a knee injury.

Equipment
A scarf, optional.

Starting Position
> Stand correctly using a wall or the back of a seat to steady yourself.

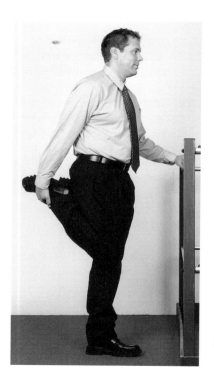

Action

> Breathe in wide, and lengthen up through the spine.
> Breathe out, zip up and hollow, and bend the right knee so you can clasp the ankle (or as far down the leg as you can comfortably reach).
> Check that you have not arched your back.
> Now, gently pull the ankle towards your buttock, keeping the knee in line with your other leg and lengthening down towards the floor. Do not take it too far back. Keep lengthening from the top of your head to your tailbone.
> Hold the stretch, breathing normally for 30 seconds or until the muscle releases.
> Repeat twice on each leg.

Side Reaches

**Warning: take advice if
you have back problems.**

Starting Position
> Stand correctly with
the feet parallel,
slightly further than
hip-width apart.

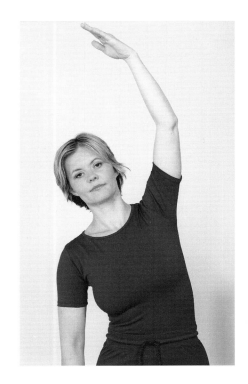

Action

> Breathe in wide.
> Breathe out, zip up and hollow. Stay zipped throughout, and float your arm up (remember Floating Arms, page 28-29).
> Rest the other hand on your outer thigh and leave it there.
> Breathe in, and lengthen up through the spine.
> Breathe out, and slowly reach across to the top corner of the room. Stretch from the waist. Keep your head and neck in line with the spine. Do not allow the pelvis to shift to one side, stay central. Try not to lean forwards or backwards – imagine that you are sliding between two doors.
> Breathe in, and return to centre.
> Lower the arm.
> Repeat five times to each side.

Calf Stretch

Starting Position

> Stand facing a wall.
> Place your hands and lower arms (with your elbows bent) against the wall.

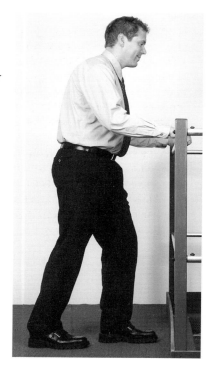

Action

> Place the toes of one leg against the base of the wall, with the feet pointing forward and the knee bent in line with the ankle.
> The opposite leg should be placed behind, in line with your hip, the leg straight, but not locked at the knee. The toes should be pointing forward and the heel down creating a stretch in the calf muscles.
> Keep the weight spread evenly through the feet between the big toe, small toe and heel.
> Keep the breathing relaxed and even, as you hold the stretch for about 20 seconds. Keep lengthening upwards. Keep zipping and hollowing.

Waist Twist

Warning: take advice if you have back problems.

Starting Position
> Stand correctly – see page 20.
> Fold your arms so that the top arm is resting lightly on the arm beneath, creating a rectangular shape. Your arms should be just above your waist, shoulder blades down into your back, upper shoulders relaxed.

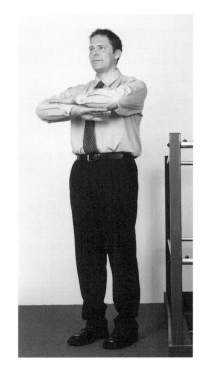

Action

> Breathe in, and lengthen up through the spine.
> Breathe out, and zip up and hollow. Staying zipped throughout and keeping your pelvis square and facing forward, gently turn your upper body around as far as is comfortable. Your head turns with your body. Only go as far as you can, keep your pelvis square and still.
> Breathe in as you return to centre.
> Repeat up to ten times to each side.

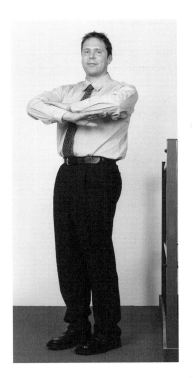

Dumb Waiter

Starting Position
> Stand correctly – see page 20.
> Hold your arms at an angle of 90° to your body, palms facing
  upwards, your elbows tucked into your waist.

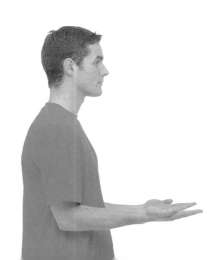

Action

> Breathe in wide, and lengthen up through the spine.
> Breathe out, zip up and hollow, and stay zipped throughout.
> Breathe in and, keeping your elbows into your sides, move your hands outwards.
> Keep the shoulders blades down so that you work the muscles between them.
> Breathe out, and return the hands to the Starting Position.
> Repeat five times.

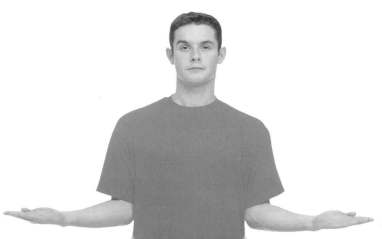

Triceps Stretch

Equipment
You may need a scarf.

Starting Position
> Stand correctly – see
page 20.
> Place one hand on the
back of your head, at
the top of your spine,
the other hand at the
base of the spine.
> Keep a sense of
openness in the front of
your body, but do not
allow the back to arch.

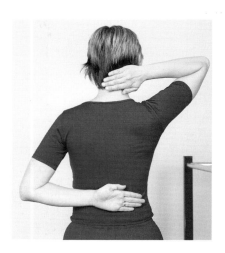

Action

> Breathe in wide, and lengthen up through the spine.
> Breathe out, zip up and hollow. Staying zipped throughout, start tracing the bones of your spine with your fingers until both hands meet. Quite probably, they will not be able to meet – please do not force them! You can use the scarf to help bring the hands together.
> Do not allow your upper back to arch.
> Take two deep breaths, keeping your head central and your ribs wide.
> Breathe out, and slowly trace your spine as you take your arms back to the Starting Position.
> Repeat three times on each side. It is common for one side to be less flexible than the other.

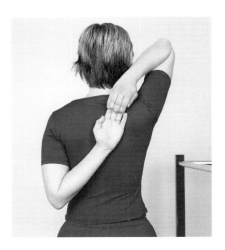

Advice upon arrival

Y OU HAVE ARRIVED! It will be a relief to stretch your legs again, so make the most of it and walk as much as you can. If possible, a gentle swim would also be beneficial.

Getting over jet lag

If you have followed all our advice for pre- and in-flight, you should be feeling fresh, but your body will still have to adjust to the new time zone. As air travel becomes faster, our bodies have found it impossible to keep up. Jet lag can cause malaise, digestive problems and, of course, tiredness – less of a worry if you are going on holiday, as you will have plenty of time to relax, but very frustrating if you have an important business meeting planned. Jet lag can reduce our decision-making skills by up to 50 per cent, and our communication skills by 30 per cent.

There are so many factors involved in jet lag. Most obvious of these are the length of the flight, the number of time zones you have crossed and whether you are arriving in the morning, afternoon or evening. If you are going to be away for just a few days it may be better to keep your body clock on home time. That is, keep meal times and sleep periods as close as possible to your usual time. Ideally, advice should be personally tailored to each traveller and their needs, but regrettably this is beyond the scope of this book. However, we can give you some general tips and advice:

> Drink plenty of water on the flight for comfort.
> You may wish to take short naps (45 minutes) to keep you on track. However, if you have travelled all night and have arrived early in the morning, go straight to your hotel room, do a few simple gentle wind-down exercises (see pages 88-95), then try to sleep for a couple of hours and no more. If you need to take an extra nap in the afternoon limit it to 45 minutes.
> Control your intake of caffeine, alcohol and tobacco within three to four hours of going to bed.
> You might think that a few alcoholic drinks will help you relax and sleep better, but in fact the opposite is true and alcohol actually disrupts sleep.
> Avoid taking too much vigorous exercise before bed – however, the gentle stretches and exercises on pages 88-95 will unwind you rather than stimulate you.
> A gentle swim, if possible, will help you relax and work your muscles at the same time.
> If you are staying in a hotel, request a quiet room.
> Hang the Do Not Disturb sign on the door.
> Tell reception to hold your calls.
> Turn off your mobile. Remember that people at home may not know you

are abroad.
> Draw the curtains and/or wear an eye mask.
> Go through your normal bedtime routine.
> It is better to be cool than to overheat; you can always keep an extra
  blanket handy in case you get cold later on.
> Schedule important meetings for your wider awake times. Remember that
  your body is programmed to be more sleepy between 3–5 a.m. and
  3–5 p.m body time.
> Use caffeine to your advantage, to wake you up when you need to
  be alert.
> Keep food simple. Avoid heavy, complicated meals that may overload
  your digestive system.

Driving exercises and advice

In addition to the known risk of DVT from prolonged sitting, driving
can also aggravate or cause back and neck problems because it
involves being seated in a fixed position often for long periods of time.
Add to this the stress of driving in heavy traffic or with restless young
children in the back seat and it is not surprising that you ache all over!

If you do suffer from back problems you might benefit from the
following advice when choosing a car:

> Ask to test drive a new car before you buy it for at least one hour to see if it is comfortable for you.
> Make sure the seat provides firm support beneath your buttocks and in the small of the back.
> If possible opt for seats that have an adjustable low-back support both in terms of the size and the height of the support. This is great because everyone's back is different and you can alter the support to suit you.
> If the seat does not have adjustable lumbar support then you may need to buy your own back support or posture wedge, or both.
> Look to see if the pedals are central, they should not be positioned off to one side or you will be driving in a twisted position.
> Power steering and an automatic gearbox will help reduce the strain on your back.
> The head restraint should not be so big that it alters your correct head/back alignment.
> If you know you will be lifting heavy luggage, etc. into the boot then choose a car with a low boot sill.

Safe journey

Before you set off:
> Plan your route carefully. Contact the AA or RAC for advice on the best routes which avoid traffic jams and roadworks. Try to familiarize yourself

with the route before you leave. Have an alternative way planned in case there are problems. Plan to stop every two hours or sooner if you are tired for at least 15 to 20 minutes, see below.

> Make sure that your car is fit for a long journey – check tyre pressures, lights, windscreen wipers and all fluid levels.
> Visit the Royal Society for the Prevention of Accidents website www.RoSPA.co.uk for safer journey planning. According to their research thousands of accidents each year are caused by tired drivers who are less alert and have less concentration. Crashes are most likely to happen:
>> on long journeys on monotonous roads, such as motorways
>> between 3.00 p.m. and 5.00 p.m. (especially after eating, or drinking even just one drink)
>> after having less sleep than usual
>> after drinking alcohol
>> after taking medicines which cause drowsiness
>> on journeys home after night shifts
> Get a good night's sleep before your journey. Avoid a long drive after a full day or night shift.
> Consider sharing the driving with someone else.
> Avoid all alcohol. Alcohol stays in the blood for several hours so you may still be affected the morning after you have had a drink.
> If you are taking medication, check to see if it causes drowsiness.
> Think about breaking up the journey with an overnight stop. If you have

an early flight to catch or if you arrive late at night – treat yourself to a hotel.

> Try the pre-trip exercises on pages 30-47 to help stretch you out before you begin.

En route

> Take plenty of still water with you.
> If you feel at all sleepy, STOP and TAKE A BREAK. Winding down the window, and turning up the radio will only work for a short while. You must stop! Caffeine (in particular strong coffee) coupled with a short nap, is especially good at keeping you alert but is no substitute for a proper rest.
> Once out of the car, don't just sit in the café, get moving. The most important exercises to do are:

Walking on the Spot page 64.

Up and Down on page 66.

> When you have done these then you can try the In Transit exercises on pages 69-81. Don't forget also that walking is excellent exercise.
> Remember all the good sitting directions given on pages 54-55.
> Try not to twist around awkwardly to get to the children (or mother-in-law!) in the back seat. Stop the car and get out to deal with them.
> Take great care when lifting small children into and out of car seats. Try

to avoid bending, twisting and lifting at the same time.

> If you are a passenger or even if you are the driver and you know you are going to be stationary for a while, then practise the following exercises to improve your circulation and keep your joints mobile:

Ankle Circles page 57
Calf Exercise page 58
Shoulder Circles page 60

Exercises for when you have reached your destination

TRAVELLING CAN BE very tiring. Whether you have travelled by air, train, coach or whether you have been driving yourself your body will feel the effects of having been in a confined space for a long period.

Allthough you will probably be anxious to rest, a few moments spent exercising now will ensure that when you wake, you will feel terrific.

If you are in a hotel room, you are unlikely to have an exercise mat with you but you can try folding the bedspread carefully or asking for a few extra bath towels. Use one underneath you, the other can be folded and used as a substitute pillow.

The following short session includes some repeats of the exercises recommended pre-flight and in transit which you will find on the pages listed below. If you have time for a longer session, you could include all the pre-flight exercises plus Walking on the Spot (page 64) and Up and Down (page 66).

Stretches (repeat pages 70-81).
Scapular Squeeze (page 90).
Corkscrew (repeat page 40).
Shoulder Drops (page 92).
Neck Rolls (repeat page 62).
Ankle Circles / Point / Flex (page 93).
Hamstring Stretch (repeat page 36).
Side-lying Quadriceps Stretch (repeat page 38).
Diamond Press (repeat page 44).
The Cat (page 94).
Rest Position (repeat page 46).

Scapular Squeeze

Starting Position
> Stand with your feet parallel and hip-width apart. Bend your knees directly over your feet.
> Pivot forward on your hips as if you are skiing downhill – your head, neck and back remain in line. Look at a spot on the floor in front of you at a distance that keeps the back of your neck free from tension and the top of the head lengthening away (see photo).
> Take your arms behind you to the sides, the palms face upwards.

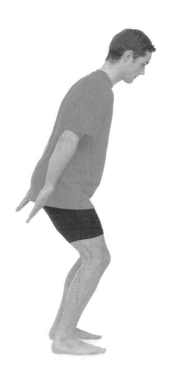

Action

> Breathe in, and lengthen through the spine.
> Breathe out, zip up and hollow and stay zipped throughout. Slide your shoulder blades down before squeezing them together.
> Your arms are also squeezing towards each other as if the thumbs want to meet.
> Breathe in.
> Breathe out, and release the arms.
> Repeat five times before returning to upright.
> When coming back to an upright position, keep lengthening your back and head away and return to a balanced way of standing, without locking your knees.

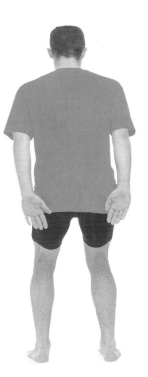

Shoulder Drops

Starting Position
> Lie in the Relaxation Position.

Action
> Raise both arms towards the ceiling directly above your shoulders, palms facing each other.
> Reach for the ceiling with one arm, stretching through the fingertips. The shoulder blade comes off the floor. Then drop the arm back down on to the floor.
> Repeat ten times with each arm, breathing normally.
> Feel your upper back widening and the tension in your shoulders releasing down into the floor.

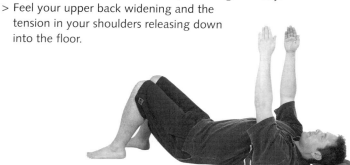

Ankle Circles / Point / Flex

Starting Position
> Lie in the Relaxation Position.
> Bend one knee up and take hold of it just above the knee.

Action
> Slowly start to circle the foot around very, very slowly, taking it as far as you can. The leg should stay completely still, the movement comes only from the ankle joint. Do not just wiggle your toes around!
> Do five circles each way.
> When you have finished the circles, point your foot away from you. Then flex the foot towards you, lengthening through the heel.
> Repeat ten times, keeping the foot in a line with your hips.

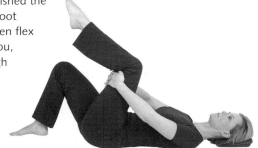

The Cat

Following this exercise, you will be coming back into the Rest Position, so have a pillow handy.

Starting Position
> Kneel on all fours, following the instructions on page 24.

Action
> Breathe in wide, lengthen through the spine.
> Breathe out, zip up and hollow. Stay zipped throughout and, starting with the base of the spine, begin to curl your tailbone under. Work your way up the back, rounding it, but keeping it

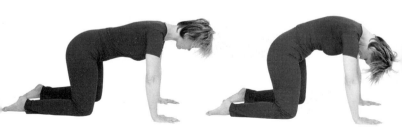

open and wide. Your chin will end up towards your chest, neck and head released. Imagine a hook pulling you from your lower back up to the ceiling.

> Breathe in wide, checking that your elbows haven't locked.
> Breathe out, and slowly uncurl, starting as before from the base of the spine. Lengthen your tailbone away, mobilizing vertebra by vertebra. Slide the shoulder blades down into your back, until you have returned to the neutral Starting Position.
> Repeat five times, taking care not to lift the head or dip the low back.
> If your wrists tire, stop for a short break, then start again. They will eventually strengthen.

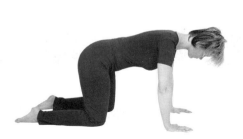

When you have finished, follow the directions for coming back into Rest Position on page 46.

Further Information

Body Control Pilates in the UK and Europe. For details of your nearest qualified Body Control Pilates teacher in the UK or Europe, please send a stamped addressed envelope to:
The Body Control Pilates Association
PO Box 29061
London
WC2H 9DZ
England

For Body Control Pilates books, videos, home equipment, teacher training courses and Pilates events, please visit the Body Control Pilates website at www.bodycontrol.co.uk

You can also write to the Body Control Pilates Association at the above address.

Body Control Pilates in North America and other countries www.bodycontrolpilates.com

Recommended Immunization

The Department of Health maintain a very comprehensive website giving advice and recommendations on health advice for travellers. www.doh.gov.uk/traveladvice

General travel advice

British Airways offer comprehensive advice regarding well being and the traveller including detailed recommendations for helping to manage the effects of jet lag. This can be found on their website at www.britishairways.com/health

For the BA travel clinics go to www.britishairways.com/travelclinic

Royal Society for the Prevention of Accidents has a website, www.RoSPA.co.uk which offers advice for safer journey planning.

Available from all good bookshops:

■ Body Control the Pilates Way
0 330 36945 8 £7.99 Pan Books
■ The Mind-Body Workout
0 330 36946 6 £12.99 Pan Books
■ Pilates the Way Forward
0 330 37081 2 £12.99 Pan Books
■ PILATES THROUGH THE DAY:
The Morning Energizer 0 330 37327 7 £2.99 Pan Books
The Desk Reviver 0 330 37328 5 £2.99 Pan Books

The Evening Relaxer 0 330 37329 3 £2.99 Pan Books
Off to Sleep 0 330 37330 7 £2.99 Pan Books
■ The Official Body Control Pilates Manual
0 330 39327 8 £12.99 Pan Books
■ Pilates Gym
0 330 48309 9 £12.99 Pan Books
■ The Body Control Pilates Back Book
0 330 48311 0 £9.99 Pan Books
■ Intelligent Exercise with Pilates & Yoga
0 333 98952 X £16.99 Macmillan

Watch out for...

■ The Perfect Body the Pilates Way
0 333 90752 3 £16.99 Macmillan November 2002

Book Services By Post, PO Box 29, Douglas, Isle of Man IM99 IBQ. Credit card hotline 01624 675 137. Postage and packing free in the UK.